# Leaky Gut Syndrome for Beginners

## - *The self-help book* -

How to correctly interpret the symptoms of a leaky gut, identify the causes and heal your gut step by step

Christoph Beckonert

# CONTENT

# What awaits you

Anyone confronted with the diagnosis of "leaky gut syndrome" will probably quickly realize during their own research that the subject is relatively complex. But why is that actually the case?

The term "leaky gut syndrome" refers to a condition in which the mucous membrane of our intestines is permeable at the microscopic level, but unfortunately not only for nutrients and other molecules important for bodily functions, but also for substances that should actually have been excreted with bowel movements, including, for example, pathogens and toxins such as alcohol. If these substances pass through the intestinal mucosa, they are then absorbed into the circulation through our blood. Our body reacts to this primarily with inflammatory reactions, which can lead to a variety of complaints.

In this guide, you will find detailed information about the structure of our digestive tract, especially the intestines, the causes and consequences of leaky gut syndrome, and information on how to diagnose it. But the most important question is actually: How do I get it under control again? The treatment of leaky gut syndrome is based primarily on three pillars: a change in diet, the reduction of stress and the rebuilding of the microbiome in the gut. In addition, there is a detailed chapter on so-called differential diagnoses, i.e. clinical pictures and complaints that lead to similar or the same symptoms but have other underlying causes and therefore need to be treated differently. Differential diagnoses of leaky gut syndrome are, for example, histamine intolerance or irritable bowel syndrome, both of which cause almost identical symptoms in those affected.

Through detailed information on the topic of nutrition and intestinal health and with the help of additional tips on stress management, you will

receive the ideal basis with which you can alleviate the symptoms of leaky gut syndrome or even
make them disappear completely. Doesn't sound
so bad, does it?

# What is a "leaky gut" anyway?

Well, first of all, it is important to know that Leaky Gut is not a recognized diagnosis of conventional medicine. The topic of leaky gut can rather be classified in the field of alternative medicine, but contrary to the assertion of some, this does not mean that leaky gut is made-up frippery. Currently, there is no evidence-based basis for the assumption that a permeable intestine is the cause of diseases such as neurodermatitis and rheumatism, or permanent complaints such as diarrhea and fatigue. However, the fact that the intestinal wall can be permeable is also known in orthodox medicine and is the case, for example, with Crohn's disease or after heavy consumption of medications and alcohol. The difference between alternative and conventional medicine on the subject of leaky gut is that conventional medicine is not currently of the opinion that a permeable intestinal wall is the cause of the diseases just mentioned as examples. If you ask me, the whole thing has a bit of the question of which came first - the chicken or the egg?

But now to the actual topic. "Leaky gut" means something like "permeable intestine". Such a leaky gut can bring a long list of problems, almost like a "domino effect". As you can imagine, a leaky gut wall causes everything we take into our gastrointestinal tract to somehow get to places where it doesn't belong. In a person with an intact intestinal mucosa, these substances would just not get into the blood, but would be excreted with the bowel movements.

In leaky gut syndrome, our intestinal mucosa can no longer react appropriately to harmful substances and pathogens, such as bacteria. As a result, the mucosa becomes permeable and the pollutants mentioned above can escape from the intestine unhindered. They thus enter the circulation through our blood. Logically, the body reacts immediately to harmful substances in the circulation, and there lies the problem. The consequences of a permeable intestine are in the end allergic and inflammatory reactions, with which the body tries to fight the harmful substances.

Imagine a mason skimping on some mortar here and there while building a house. The façade leaks and it rains in. It's not quite that simple, of course, but broadly speaking, this example describes what happens in our bodies during leaky gut syndrome.

## OUR DIGESTIVE SYSTEM - AN OVERVIEW

A person's digestive tract is a very complex system and consists of many components, all of which must be well coordinated. Leaky gut syndrome occurs mainly in the large intestine, but to recognize and understand problems and diseases of the gastrointestinal tract, it is not enough to look only at the affected part.

The digestion of our food begins in the mouth and not, as is often mistakenly assumed, in the stomach. After ingestion of food through the mouth, the food is broken down with the help of our teeth and tongue. In addition, the mouth is supplied with saliva, which is produced in the salivary glands. During the chewing process, this is mixed with the food pulp. Our saliva contains the so-called amylase, which is an enzyme that breaks down carbohydrates into sugars. If you chew a piece of bread well and keep it in your mouth for a while before swallowing, you may have noticed that the bread quickly begins to taste sweet. It is at this point that you notice how amylase breaks down the carbohydrates in the bread into sugars. Through the pharynx, the food passes into the esophagus and from there into the stomach. In the stomach, the gastric glands produce about two liters of digestive secretion, gastric juice, per day. It consists mainly of hydrochloric acid, which is, however, very diluted in the stomach. In addition, the gastric juice contains the enzyme pepsin, which can cleave proteins, and the so-called intrinsic factor. This intrinsic factor is used for the absorption of vitamin B12 in the small intestine.

The duodenum then joins the stomach like a tube and is also called the duodenum. Ducts from the pancreas, the pancreas and the gallbladder flow into the duodenum, enriching the small intestine with further digestive secretions. The secretion from the pancreas contains further enzymes for the cleavage of carbohydrates, proteins, fats, cholesterol and nucleic acids, such as DNA and RNA. The secretion from the bile contains mainly bile acids, which are mainly used for digestion and utilization of fats. By the way, the liquid of bile is produced in the liver, the gallbladder serves only to store this liquid. The duodenum is then followed by the rest of the small intestine, whose function is to break down and utilize nutrients. The small intestine is followed by the large intestine. The large intestine is mainly responsible for the absorption of water from the food pulp, thus thickening it. The large intestine is much more heavily colonized by bacteria than the small intestine. To prevent the bacteria and the food pulp from passing back from the large intestine into the small intestine, the two are separated from each other by a kind of valve. After the large intestine, the stool enters the rectum and is excreted from there.

## THE INTESTINE AS PART OF THE IMMUNE SYSTEM

Our intestine, or gastrointestinal tract, is a huge organ. It lies entwined in our abdominal cavity in a very small space, but can reach a total length of seven or eight meters. That's quite a lot, don't you think?

But that is not enough. In order to absorb as many nutrients as possible from our food, our intestines need as large an area as possible. The absorption of nutrients through our intestines is called resorption. Since there is not an infinite amount of space in the human body, nature has come up with something else to increase the surface area. Microscopically, our intestines consist of millions of so-called villi and crypts. These are microscopic elevations and depressions of our intestinal mucosa. Imagine a landscape in which there are always alternating mountains and valleys, and millions of them. Due to this construction, our intestine is able to cover a huge area in a very small space, namely almost 400 square meters. That corresponds to almost an entire basketball court!

Seen in cross-section, our intestine consists of 3 layers. The innermost, which comes into direct contact with food, is a layer of mucus, also called the mucosa. It consists of enterocytes, i.e. the typical cells of the intestine, and also contains a particularly large amount of lymphatic tissue in the form of microscopic lymph follicles. These serve the immune defense. In the middle lies a layer of muscle, which once again consists of two layers, a ring muscle layer and a longitudinal muscle layer. This keeps the intestine in motion and allows it to transport food through contractions. This is also called peristalsis. The outermost layer is called adventitia or serosa, depending on its position in the abdominal cavity; it separates the intestine from the abdominal cavity and consists mainly of connective tissue. The individual cells of the intestine are connected to each other by so-called tight junctions, which are protein complexes that hold the cell association in place.

Another very important part of our intestines is the microbiome, also known as intestinal flora. The term intestinal flora is somewhat erroneous, however, as the co-inhabitants in our intestines are of course not plants, so I will not use it further here. Most bacteria of our microbiome are found in the large intestine on the mucus layer, i.e. the innermost layer. It is estimated that up to 1,000 different types of bacteria live on the walls of our intestines, and the weight of them is estimated at almost 1.5 kilograms! That seems like a lot, but when you think about how many tasks these organisms perform for us, it explains a lot.

The bacteria in our intestines break down carbohydrates and proteins, produce vitamins, neutralize pollutants and serve as an immune defense. Bacteria usually have a rather bad image, as we often associate them with diseases or infections. However, it is not quite that simple, let's take a closer look. The bacteria that benefit us, for example by producing vitamins or aiding digestion by splitting large molecules, usually live with us in a symbiosis or as commensals. Symbiosis means that host (human) and parasite (bacterium) both benefit from each other, because the bacteria support our nutrient supply and the human provides the bacterium with a place where it can optimally multiply and grow. In other words, a win-win situation. Commensals, on the other hand, are organisms that receive an advantage from the host but neither benefit nor harm it. However, they can become pathogenic, i.e. trigger a disease or cause discomfort. This happens, for example, after a person has taken antibiotics for a long period of time, because antibiotics, as the name suggests, inhibit or kill bacteria. I'll explain how to rebalance the gut after taking antibiotics in a later post. And now enough about the anatomy of our intestines. Much more important is what this "leaky gut" is all about.

## HOW DOES THE LEAKY GUT DEVELOP?

Exactly what causes the intestinal wall to become permeable is not yet entirely clear and probably depends on several factors. For example, the mucosa and microbiome may be attacked, hindering the immune response. It is also possible that the tight junctions, i.e. the connection between the cells, are destroyed or loosened, so that harmful substances can more easily "migrate" between the gaps created.

It is suspected that certain toxins, for example alcohol, nicotine and drugs such as cortisone, trigger leaky gut syndrome. However, it is also possible that certain foods can lead to leaky gut. Currently, sugar and white flour are suspected, but also fermented foods such as tofu or soy sauce. Permanent stress and an unhealthy lifestyle, for example through little exercise, can also promote the development of leaky gut syndrome. Also negative for intestinal health are cytostatics, which are drugs used in the treatment of cancer through chemotherapy, as they inhibit cell division and have a very aggressive effect. That is why patients undergoing treatment with chemotherapeutic agents often also experience additional intestinal problems. Basically, anything that is unhealthy anyway is conducive to leaky gut.

# CONSEQUENCES OF A LEAKY GUT

As I have already touched on, substances enter our blood and circulation through the permeable intestinal wall that actually do not belong there. The body defends itself against this by trying to render the harmful substances harmless through allergic and inflammatory reactions. This can lead to many different symptoms, the variety of which makes it difficult to clearly identify them with leaky gut syndrome. For example, affected individuals may suffer from pain in joints and muscles, as well as concentration problems, acne, neurodermatitis, fatigue, skin redness, itching, severe abdominal pain and diarrhea.

A study by Smith et al. in the Journal of Rheumatology showed as early as the 1980s that patients with rheumatic diseases had increased permeability in their intestinal mucosa. Another study by Swedish researchers at Malmö University in 2014 showed that patients suffering from multiple sclerosis had leaky gut long before.

There are various ways to diagnose leaky gut syndrome. However, because the symptoms are so varied and rather non-specific, the path to the correct diagnosis is usually long.

One diagnostic option is the lactulose-mannitol test. Lactulose is a sugar consisting of two different sugar molecules, while mannitol is a sugar alcohol. A mixture of lactulose and mannitol is administered to the patient, and urine and blood can then be tested for the two substances a few hours later. A conspicuous lactulose-mannitol test can indicate leaky gut syndrome.

Furthermore, there is the possibility to test the level of zonulin in the blood or in the stool. Zonulin is a protein that can be secreted by the mucosa in the intestine. It is believed that zonulin increases the permeability of the intestinal mucosa by relaxing the tight junctions. However, this is currently still a theory and has not been conclusively researched. In theory, therefore, elevated zonulin levels may also be an indication of leaky gut. This test is criticized for not doing justice to the complexity of the intestinal mucosa and its function in nutrient utilization, because it oversimplifies the physiological processes in the intestine. Currently, the Zonulin test is not covered by most statutory health insurers. Both tests have been criticized and are not conclusive on the basis of test results alone. A diagnosis should never consist of only one test, but should always be made additionally by a detailed anamnesis, a physical examination and by cause research. This applies not only to leaky gut syndrome, but actually to all clinical pictures.

There are many self-tests for leaky gut syndrome on the Internet. Some offer tests that are supposed to be easy to perform at home, while others allow you to send stool samples, for example, which are then examined in a laboratory. I would like to advise you against such dubious offers. Such tests are usually incredibly expensive and not worth the money, because they make some kind of diagnosis without knowing the patient's background story. They are definitely not meaningful and can in no way replace a consultation with a doctor.

# Leaky gut and histamine intolerance

Histamine - ever heard of it? Histamine is a hormone in the human body, it consists of a kind of modification of the basic amino acid histidine. It is produced, among other things, by the so-called mast cells, which are found primarily in the skin and in the gastrointestinal tract. They play an important role in allergic processes in particular, because they can recognize antigens and react accordingly. But we can also absorb large amounts of histamines through food, more on this later. In the gastrointestinal tract, they react on contact with pathogenic substances, for example by increasing the release of fluid into the intestine and peristalsis.

This can lead to diarrhea and faster digestion and elimination of harmful substances. Histamine is broken down in the body by diamine oxidase, or DAO or histaminase for short. The functions of histamine are manifold and very different, depending on which organ it is acting on. In the stomach, histamine increases the secretion of gastric acid. In the circulatory system, it can dilate or constrict vessels, thus affecting blood circulation. In addition, histamine can cause the smooth muscles in our bronchial tubes to contract. Smooth muscles are muscles that humans cannot control at will, so the bronchial tubes can become constricted and breathing problems, such as in asthma, can be the result. Every person can tolerate a certain amount of histamine well, but if more histamine is ingested, allergic reactions occur, for example itching, reddening of the skin, wheals, shortness of breath, diarrhea and severe abdominal pain.

So much for histamine in general - now I would like to go into more detail about histamine intolerance. In histamine intolerance, the amount of histamine that a person can consume without problems is significantly reduced. The symptoms just mentioned in case of a histamine "overdose" occur much faster in intolerant people. The cause of an intolerance to histamine is usually a deficiency or malfunction of diamine oxidase, i.e. the substance that is actually supposed to break down histamine. Thus histamine accumulates in the body and an allergic reaction occurs.

Unfortunately, there is currently no therapy for histamine intolerance, but the symptoms can be significantly alleviated by a low-histamine diet. The intake of diamine oxidase, i.e. the enzyme that is missing in histamine-intolerant people, is currently not an alternative to a low-histamine diet, since studies have not yet been able to prove a positive effect. In general, it can be said that the histamine content increases in foods that have been matured, stored and fermented for a long time. Foods that contain a lot of histamine and should therefore be avoided are, for example:

• Meat in the form of sausage, cold cuts, salami, etc.

• Salted and dried fish and seafood

• Cheese (especially more matured varieties, for example Parmesan)

• Red wine

• Fermented, for example, tofu and soy sauce

• Tomatoes, eggplant, spinach

• Kiwis, strawberries, citrus fruits

• Cocoa and chocolate

• Lemons and strawberries (strictly speaking, these do not contain very much histamine, but they do cause a release of histamine in the mast cells and should therefore be avoided).

This may sound as if you are not allowed to eat anything if you have a histamine intolerance. Of course, this is not the case. I would like to emphasize here that it is about eating low in histamine and not histamine-free. Histamine-intolerant people tolerate a certain amount of histamine, but less than others. To give you a complete list of low-histamine foods would go too far here. There are countless lists on the Internet that you can use to orient yourself well and in detail. Foods that contain little histamine and can usually be eaten without any problems include:

• Meat and fish in unprocessed and not preserved form

• Milk, cream cheese, cottage cheese

• Chia seeds, psyllium seeds, flax seeds, coconut, pistachios, pumpkin seeds

• Many types of vegetables and fruits, for example, blueberries, apples, mangoes, melons, cucumber, broccoli, potatoes, carrots and some others.

There is currently no gold standard for diagnosing histamine intolerance. Tests to measure the concentration of histamine or diamine oxidase in the blood are not recommended, as they have not yet proven to be conclusive. However, there is the possibility of a prick test, here a small prick is placed in the skin and sprinkled with histamine. In the case of intolerance, wheals usually form on the affected area. If these do not disappear after 50 minutes, it can be assumed that the skin cannot properly break down the histamine.

However, this test does not mean that histamine, which was taken in through food, cannot be broken down properly either. Therefore, this test is also not completely reliable. The most sensible thing to do here is also to observe your body. Do you often have itching, reddening of the skin, diarrhea, stomach pain, headaches or similar, rather unspecific symptoms after meals that contained a lot of histamine? Then one possible explanation is definitely histamine intolerance. If you reduce the intake of histamine through food and the symptoms also reduce quickly, the matter is clear relatively quickly.

You are probably wondering what all this has to do with leaky gut syndrome. The symptoms of both are relatively similar and unspecific, and in addition, a diagnosis by a simple test is not always conclusive, so that in both histamine intolerance and leaky gut syndrome, observation and appropriate changes in diet achieve the greatest success. Of course, a person can potentially suffer from both at the same time, so both should always be considered for the symptoms mentioned.

# Leaky Gut and Irritable Bowel

Irritable bowel syndrome, or IBS, is an unpleasant thing. Perhaps you have already heard of it. Sufferers of irritable bowel syndrome suffer from severe discomfort of the gastrointestinal tract. This includes diarrhea, bloating, constipation and severe abdominal pain. Although IBS is not a dangerous disease, sufferers can suffer greatly, psychologically and physically. The symptoms of irritable bowel syndrome worsen greatly with stress in a large proportion of sufferers. How exactly or why irritable bowel syndrome develops is currently not entirely clear, but similar changes in the intestine are found in many sufferers.

Firstly, the peristalsis of the intestine is often disturbed, i.e. the contractions with which the intestine moves the food. Peristalsis is controlled by the autonomic nervous system, the part of our nervous system that we cannot control voluntarily. If our colon receives the "wrong" information from the autonomic nervous system, for example, it contracts too slowly, the food remains in the colon too long and this can cause constipation and abdominal pain. The main function of our large intestine is the absorption of water from the food pulp, so it is thickened. However, if the intestine contracts too quickly, the food does not remain in the colon long enough and not enough water can be absorbed. This can lead to diarrhea.

In addition, people suffering from irritable bowel syndrome often have an increased permeability of the mucous membrane in the intestine. You understand what I am getting at?

In irritable bowel patients, it has been observed that tight junctions break down too quickly. You may recall, tight junctions were the protein complexes that firmly connect the cells of the intestinal mucosa. If there are not enough junctions, or if the existing junctions are not tight enough, the intestinal mucosa becomes permeable. Furthermore, it was found that irritable bowel patients have an increased number of immune and defense cells in the intestine and they often also have a disturbed microbiome in the intestine.

Unfortunately, as with leaky gut syndrome, it is relatively difficult to diagnose irritable bowel syndrome. Therefore, it is usually a diagnosis of exclusion. This refers to diagnoses that can only be assumed after the doctor has been able to rule out all other causes for the symptoms. For example, allergies and intolerance to food can also be the cause of diarrhea and abdominal pain, such a reason for the complaints should always be excluded. Diagnostically, the three typical "craft skills" of a physician should be used above all: Percussion, palpation and auscultation, i.e. tapping, palpation and listening. By examining the tapping sound on the abdomen, it is possible to find out whether and to what extent the intestine is filled with air or stool.

By palpating, the person treating the patient can see whether the patient has thickening or tension in certain parts of the intestine and whether a feeling of pain can be triggered there by palpation. In addition, by listening with a stethoscope, the peristalsis, i.e. activity and movement, of the intestines can be determined. Finally, a blood test can determine whether inflammation is present. A typical inflammation value in the blood is the so-called CRP, which means C-reactive protein. The CRP value rises in the case of inflammation and can thus quickly provide indications of inflammatory processes in the body. In healthy people, the normal value of C-reactive protein is about 5 mg per liter. It is important to note, however, that the CRP level increases with almost any type of inflammatory process in the body, for example, even with a cold, so it is not limited to inflammation in the intestines. The cause of an elevated CRP level should therefore always be investigated by further tests.

The DGVS, i.e. the German Society for Digestive and Metabolic Diseases, specifies that at least three of the following criteria must be met for a diagnosis of irritable bowel syndrome: severe impairment of quality of life due to the bowel complaints, the complaints cannot be caused by the presence of similar diseases, the complaints are persistent and occur at least once a week.

It is very important for me to say that fever, severe weight loss and blood in the stool, for example, are not associated with IBS. Such symptoms can have their origin in serious diseases of the gastrointestinal tract and should be clarified by a doctor in any case!

Unfortunately, irritable bowel syndrome can currently only be treated symptomatically. This means that the treatment does not combat the cause, but "only" the resulting problems. Since the symptoms can vary greatly among those affected and range from diarrhea to constipation, the therapy should always be adapted to the individual patient. As already mentioned, stress greatly aggravates the symptoms in most sufferers. Stress should therefore be avoided as far as possible, more on this in the chapter "Reducing stress". In addition, foods to which the body reacts by aggravating the symptoms should be avoided. For example, beans are known to cause constipation and flatulence. Coffee and spicy foods or spices, on the other hand, cause diarrhea or abdominal pain in many people, especially those with a sensitive stomach or intestines.

To alleviate the symptoms, non-drug therapies, such as a reduction in stress and a change in diet, should be the first choice. However, if symptoms persist, the use of medications should also be considered. Depending on the symptoms, this could be painkillers, antidiarrheals or laxative medications, for example. However, the use of medications should always be clarified by a doctor, especially if the drugs are taken permanently or very often. They can lead to severe side effects if they are not dosed correctly or are contraindicated!

Many people shy away from taking medication, especially when the complaints are rather "mild". In principle, of course, it is not sensible to take paracetamol or ibuprofen for every little ache, that is probably clear. For example, ibuprofen and paracetamol are metabolized in the liver and cause liver damage. No effect without a side effect, as the saying goes. However, it is still very important to understand two things. First, there are no prizes for being brave, at least not for most adults. Unfortunately, if you lie on the couch or in bed all day with aches and pains, no one will thank you in the end. People with chronic diseases tend, especially at the beginning of their diagnosis, to be ashamed of their complaints and to limit their social life because of the discomfort. This kind of behavior over the long term can lead not only to physical complaints but also to psychological problems.

Secondly, permanent pain and discomfort can cause us to adopt a protective posture. In the case of bone fractures or damage to muscles and tendons, a protective posture can greatly worsen the healing process. Because of the reduced load, the affected area receives less blood flow and movement than the healthy side. In addition, this creates imbalances and incorrect strain on muscles, which can lead to pain. Something like this can also happen with a protective posture due to intestinal complaints, for example, if the affected person lies down a lot or assumes a hunched posture. So there is nothing to be said against taking medication in a medically approved and responsible manner.

Mentioning irritable bowel syndrome and histamine intolerance in this reading was important to me because both can be differential diagnoses in relation to leaky gut syndrome. Differential diagnoses are diseases or diagnoses that have very similar symptoms to the suspected disease. In medicine, it is very important to always keep possible differential diagnoses in mind as well, because the therapy may be completely different for the same symptoms. In order to be able to distinguish the differential diagnoses from each other, it is therefore very important to place a special focus on the causes of the complaints.

# And what can I do myself now?

First of all, you can breathe a sigh of relief. Having leaky gut syndrome is really not pleasant, but fortunately, leaky gut is relatively easy to treat. The three most important components of treatment are a change in diet, reduction of stress levels in everyday life and supportive treatment with probiotics.

Another piece of good news for you: The intestinal mucosa has a very high mitosis rate compared to the rest of the body. The mitotic rate indicates how fast the cells in the body divide, i.e. also regenerate. This means that with the right dietary changes and treatment, you may notice a rapid improvement in symptoms.

## CHANGE DIET

In the treatment of leaky gut syndrome, it is first of all indispensable to question one's own diet and then to change it in a needs-oriented manner. What exactly I mean by "needs-oriented" I will explain in more detail later.

It is anything but sensible to simply eliminate foods such as white flour, sugar and fermented foods from one's diet overnight. It is much more important to first learn to observe and understand your own eating behavior and the reaction of your body. I also know that this is not so easy, but nevertheless it is very important to learn how your own body works and reacts. Observe yourself: For example, what do you eat on days when you are working and have a rather elevated stress level? How does your body react to this? Compare your diet and your body's reaction with the days when you are more relaxed. Because as mentioned earlier, stress also plays an important role in a leaky gut. Of course, it's best to note what you ate and how you felt afterwards.

Of course, you can write this down on paper the old-fashioned way, but now there are also some apps that can be used to monitor eating habits. Regardless of how you want to solve this, one thing is important above all: stay on the ball. The longer you observe yourself, the better you will be able to respond to your body's needs in the end. This can sometimes take a few weeks, maybe even a few months. But I promise you: It's worth it!

Now, if you could notice that a certain food increases the symptoms of leaky gut syndrome in you, you can start to eliminate it more and more from your daily diet. This is sometimes not so easy, I know. I'm sure most of you will quickly notice that sugar, for example, increases the symptoms of leaky gut. Unfortunately, however, it is almost impossible to eat a sugar-free diet these days. Sugar can be found, even often hidden, in countless foods. In addition, the "withdrawal" of sugar in most of us leads to strong cravings and initially also to concentration problems, so sooner or later a dissatisfaction sets in. You can find out how to recognize hidden sugars and counteract cravings through a balanced diet in the "Food Guide" chapter.



## REDUCE STRESS

Everyone knows that stress is unhealthy. Stress has a negative effect on our psyche and can lead to serious illnesses, such as depression and burnout. In the same way, stress can also affect the body physically. Many of you have probably already heard of stress-related gastritis. But how exactly does stress negatively affect our bodies, especially our intestines?

Our nervous system consists of a part that we can control ourselves, for example by actively moving our muscles, speaking and much more. Another part of our nervous system is not controllable by us voluntarily, this part is called the autonomic nervous system and it consists of the sympathetic and the parasympathetic nervous system. The parasympathetic nervous system is activated when we are in relaxed and safe situations. It controls the bodily functions that are vital for humans, but can be "switched off" in dangerous situations, because they are rather secondary in the fight for life or death. These include, for example, the feeling of hunger or the urge to go to the toilet.

Its counterpart, the sympathetic nervous system, on the other hand, releases adrenaline and cortisol when we find ourselves in dangerous situations. These two substances increase our performance and use the body's energy for vital functions, such as muscle strength, thus ensuring survival. You have probably heard of the famous "fight or flight" principle.

But what happens when we are constantly exposed to stress in everyday life? Well, the body activates the sympathetic nervous system and energy is used for functions in the body that are necessary for survival. The energy for these actions must be withdrawn from the "unnecessary" functions at that moment, for example our intestines. Thus, peristalsis, i.e. the movement of the intestines for digestion, is inhibited or even stopped completely. This can lead to complaints such as constipation or even abdominal pain. As a result, however, diarrhea can also develop, because if the intestine can no longer extract water from the food due to the energy it has been deprived of, the water remains in the excretion. Neither is very nice. In addition, adrenaline and cortisol not only affect energy distribution in the body, but also the gut microbiome, because they have a damaging effect on the bacteria that colonize our gut. If the beneficial bacteria that support digestion are inhibited, this also leads to constipation, diarrhea or abdominal pain.

So for a healthy body and a healthy gut, it's essential to keep stress levels as low as possible. Of course, this does not always work. Stress is not bad per se, as it can spur us on and protect us from threatening situations. But when stress becomes a permanent condition, it is simply not healthy. Every person has his or her own strategy for dealing with stress. Walking, meditating, meeting with friends, again, start observing yourself and learn what is good for your body.

## RESILIENCE

Resilience is a term from psychology and refers to the ability to respond to crises, overcome them and then use them for personal development. An example would be a child who grows up in a violent environment, but later leads a successful life anyway and uses the traumas of the past to pass on better values to their own children in adulthood. Another example is an adult who does not give up after a severe blow of fate or trauma, perhaps a serious accident or the death of someone close, but is able to continue his or her life.

There are various factors that can positively or negatively influence a person's resilience, as a synonym for which I would also like to use resilience here. For example, support from the social environment (friends, family, colleagues and so on), intelligence and the ability to control one's own emotions have a positive effect on resilience. Negative effects include toxic relationships (whether friendly, familial, or romantic) and a low capacity for impulse and self-control.

According to current research, resilience is partly innate. However, another part can be trained. I would now like to take a closer look at resilience training. Resilience training has been shown to have little effect on children, but it can have noticeable effects on adults. Resilience training is basically based on seven pillars:

**1. Acceptance**: Unfortunately, it sounds like that, but acceptance plays a very decisive role in coping with crises and stress. If a situation cannot be changed at that moment, then you must try to make the best of it. After all, if you dwell on it too long, you will waste your own resources.

**2. Positive thinking**: Sometimes you think to y- ourself, "today was a really bad day, just everyth- ing went wrong that could have gone wrong in any way". But was everything really bad today? On such days, there are usually two or three big things that went really badly. You should accept that and then think about whether *everything* was really bad today. Mostly, there are also some nice little things on such days, which have somehow been pushed into the background by the "bad" day. Perhaps the gas prices were particularly favorable or the person who sold you the coffee was parti- cularly friendly. Think about it.

**3. Self-perception**: Most people perceive them- selves much worse than their outside world does. We are often far too critical of ourselves because we lack the ability to assess ourselves objectively, as if from a bird's eye view. However, it is possible to train people to evaluate themselves without bias. An example: You gave an important presentation at work today. After you finish, you go home feeling like you did very poorly. Now take a metaphorical bird's eye view, in this case perhaps the perspective of a colleague who has a neutral relationship with you. What three points would this person have mentioned as praise or criticism with regard to your presentation?

**4. Optimism**: Just as we tend to see ourselves as worse than we are, we also tend to always imagine the "worst case". Then the disappointment is not so high in the end. That may be so, but the incentive to overcome this hurdle will then be just as low. What might the "best case" look like, and is it really much less likely than the worst case?

**5. Control and responsibility**: Resilient people know that they have influence over the course of certain things in their lives. Of course, this does not apply to everything in life, for example, not to a death in an acquaintance. If you are unhappy with a situation, think about how that situation could be changed for the better. Take responsibility for the things that can be influenced and do not remain in the victim role.

**6. Fellow human beings**: Resilient people usually have a large and reliable social network. Just the thought of not being alone with a problem helps many people. If you don't know what to do, talk to someone you trust about it. Being resilient doesn't mean solving all your problems on your own.

**7. Reminder**: When you are faced with a major challenge that seems impossible to overcome, try to remember: "What hurdles have I been able to overcome in the past? Before that, I felt the same way I feel right now, and yet I was able to do it. Then I can manage this one, too."

## PROBIOTICS AS A COMPLEMENTARY TREATMENT

Probiotics are not to be confused with prebiotics, which I will discuss later in the Food Guide. Probiotics are preparations of non-pathogenic, i.e. not disease-causing, living microorganisms. They usually contain bacteria, yeasts or microscopic algae. The bacteria contained in probiotics include lactobacilli. These are bacteria that can produce lactic acid from glucose through fermentation processes. Another microorganism commonly found in probiotics is yeast with the lovely name Saccharomyces boulardii, also known as "medicinal yeast." Saccharomyces boulardii is also often recommended for persistent diarrhea because this yeast secretes substances called proteases that break down toxins. It can also bind pathogens and thus render them harmless.

The mode of action of probiotics is thus ensured by various mechanisms. The organisms contained can bind pathogens, "destroy" their food or reduce the pH value, i.e. shift it to an acidic environment. In fact, most bacteria tend to grow optimally in an alkaline environment. As I mentioned earlier, antibiotics can really mess up the microbiome, which quickly leads to gastrointestinal complaints.

Here it is helpful to take probiotic preparations orally as a preventive measure after antibiotic therapy has ended in order to counteract gastrointestinal problems. It is important to take probiotics in sufficient quantities, otherwise their effectiveness is not guaranteed. Probiotic preparations are available over the counter in virtually every pharmacy, but it is still advisable to discuss their use with your doctor.

# Food guide

In the following, I have created a small guide for you, which should give you a deeper understanding of the food you encounter every day. It should make shopping in the supermarket a little easier for you. Partially I will also go into the chemical basics of the substances, but please don't let that scare you away.

Keeping track of the variety of artificial or natural ingredients in certain foods can sometimes be quite difficult. To give you the opportunity to take a closer look at foods before you put them in your shopping cart the next time you go shopping, you will find more detailed information on various substances in this chapter.

This guidebook does not consist of "10 commandments" that you must follow in order to make positive changes to your intestinal health. Everyone has a craving for cookies, cakes or chips from time to time, and that's perfectly normal and absolutely not a bad thing. However, eating a little healthier and, most importantly, *more consciously* will not only do your gut good, but the rest of your body as well. So see this guide as a kind of guide from which you are welcome to take inspiration, but without suddenly having to give up everything that is not organic and healthy.

## PREBIOTICS

Prebiotics are not the same as probiotics. I already mentioned that. By taking probiotics orally, you are taking beneficial bacteria and yeast into your body. Prebiotics, on the other hand, are effectively food for the organisms you already have inside you. In other words, they support your body's existing "resources." For example, psyllium and flaxseed are considered prebiotics.

Their effect is that they are broken down by the intestinal microbiome. This produces substances such as lactic acid, which in turn serve as food for the microbiome. In addition, short-chain fatty acids, known as carboxylic acids, such as butyric acid, are produced during the breakdown process. Acids contribute to the pH value in the intestine becoming lower, i.e. more acidic. As we have already learned, an acidic environment makes it harder for pathogens to grow. While psyllium husks and flaxseeds may not sound appealing, I promise you that incorporating them into your diet is as easy as pie. Psyllium husks and flaxseeds are small and have virtually no taste of their own. Therefore, they can be mixed very well in the morning in, for example, muesli and yogurt. You can also simply mix them into bread doughs and eat them that way. There are really a few options, feel free to try out what works best for you.

## PROTEINS

Walking the aisles of supermarkets today, one thing stands out above all else: Protein, protein, protein. Almost every food product advertises a high protein content. Yogurts, cereals, bars, even on pasta. Well, what is it actually about these proteins? Aren't they only important for people who want to build muscles in the gym? I'll say right away: No, not at all. But let's first get to what they are actually made of.

Proteins, also called proteins, consist of amino acids. There are 21 proteinogenic amino acids, i.e. amino acids that serve the body to make proteins from them. Amino acids can have different properties. In fact, they always consist of a solid basic structure, but differ from each other only in a single "appendage". Depending on the chemical properties of this appendage, the amino acid can also be acidic or basic and water-soluble or water-insoluble. Several amino acids link together with the release of some water to form a protein. The tasks of proteins in the body are manifold. They serve cell growth, accelerate physiological processes, store oxygen and much more. The daily protein requirement for adults is approximately one gram of protein per kilogram of body weight. For people who do a lot of sports and want to build up muscles, the advice is even 1.5 grams per kilogram of body weight. So you can easily calculate how much protein you need per day. More about this later.

An important concept in proteins is biological value. As already mentioned, proteins consist of several amino acids that are linked together. The more the amino acid composition of a protein resembles the body's amino acid requirements, the higher the biological value of this protein. Thus, the biological value describes how well an ingested protein can be converted into the body's own protein. Proteins consist partly of nitrogen and are the most important source of nitrogen for humans. Therefore, the biological value of a protein can be calculated based on the uptake and release of nitrogen. The protein from chicken eggs, for example, has a biological value of 100, followed by tuna, for example, with 92, cow's milk with 82 and poultry with 80. However, the biological value says nothing about the content of vitamins or other minerals and is therefore more of a guide than a measure of how healthy a food is.

Symptoms of protein deficiency include fatigue and exhaustion, hair loss, dry skin and brittle nails. Proteins are not only hidden in meat, many nuts and legumes actually contain a lot of proteins. These include peanuts, beans, chickpeas and lentils, for example. With a conscious diet, it is actually very easy to cover the daily protein requirement, even with a vegetarian or vegan diet. One important point I have kept from you until now. Proteins saturate faster than carbohydrates and, above all, they saturate for a very long time. This means that with a sufficient daily intake of proteins you can prevent cravings, which usually end with the intake of mountains of sugar. If the craving is already there, you can also fight it with a protein-rich snack, for example with nuts or a protein bar. In this way, proteins not only help you lose weight, as the long-lasting feeling of satiety means that fewer carbohydrates and calories are consumed, but they also have a positive effect on a leaky gut, as they help you eat less sugar.

## CARBOHYDRATES AND SUGAR

Carbohydrates and sugar. Some people feel a shiver down their spine just hearing these words. But that is not justified. The vast majority of foods cannot be pigeonholed as "good" or "bad" anyway and should always be viewed in a differentiated manner. Let's start, as with proteins, with the chemical basis of these two substances. Carbohydrates are made up of sugar molecules and can be categorized depending on the number of sugar molecules in their basic structure.

First of all, there are simple sugars, which, as you can already imagine, are made up of one sugar molecule. These include, for example, glucose and fructose, which, as you know, also taste sweet. Next come dual sugars, consisting of two sugar molecules. This category includes lactose, or milk sugar, and sucrose, the familiar household sugar. These two also taste sweet. Finally, there are the polysaccharides, which consist of more than two sugar molecules. The best-known representative of these is starch, which no longer tastes sweet. The different types of sugar have different properties, for example they can be utilized by the body at different rates.

The German Nutrition Society (DGE) recommends that at least 50% of the food energy per day should consist of carbohydrates - but here I have to hook in directly, the sugar content of these carbohydrates should be as small as possible. Too bad. Healthy carbohydrate sources are for example sweet potatoes, oat flakes, quinoa or legumes. Due to their additional high protein content, legumes are therefore particularly healthy.

We now know that not all sugar is the same. There are countless names for unhealthy sugars in the ingredients of foods, so it is sometimes difficult to see through where sugar is contained and where it is not. A completely sugar-free diet is certainly possible, but I personally would not recommend it. Our body needs sugar and carbohydrates to work and function. Our brain even needs a whole 140 grams of sugar per day.

I would just like to encourage you to consciously consume a little less sugar. Sugar can be found in many foods that would do well without it, for example in crispbread, bread, pesto, fruit yogurts, cream cheese, various spreads and other products. Nevertheless, there are enough alternatives that do not contain sugar and can be found quickly on the shelf if you take the time. Sugar-free alternatives by no means taste less good than the products with sugar. Most of the time, you don't even notice the difference. Also, sugar-free products are not only organic and expensive, usually the supermarket's own brand does as well.

# FAT

Surprise - fats are basically not bad either. Fats consist of fatty acids, i.e. the long-chain carboxylic acids I mentioned earlier. Chemically, fats can be distinguished from other macromolecules, such as proteins and fats, primarily by their poor solubility in water. There are apolar lipids, which do not dissolve at all or only very poorly in water, and there are amphiphilic lipids. These consist of a water-soluble part and another water-insoluble part. An example of this is the phospholipids that make up our cell membrane. The lipids we ingest through our food are usually apolar, meaning they cannot be dissolved in water. Because of their apolarity and size, they cannot be absorbed by the cells in our intestinal mucosa. That is why they have to be broken down during digestion by so-called lipases, which are enzymes, and are then packaged into water-soluble structures so that they can now be absorbed and metabolized.

The fatty acids that make up our fats can also be categorized. There are saturated, monounsaturated and polyunsaturated fatty acids. Saturated fatty acids consist only of single bonds between the carbon atoms; they can be produced by our body itself and are found, for example, in butter and palm oil. Monounsaturated fatty acids have a double bond between the carbon atoms, they can be found in olive oil and rapeseed oil, among others. Lastly, we have the polyunsaturated fatty acids, which have two or more double bonds. Particularly important representatives of this group are omega-6 and omega-3 fatty acids, this designation indicates the position of the last double bond in the molecule. Omega-3 and omega-6 fatty acids have been shown to reduce the risk of diseases of the cardiovascular system, such as heart attacks and coronary heart disease.

They are essential, which means that our body cannot produce them itself and therefore we have to take them in with food. Ideally, omega-6 and omega-3 should be consumed in a ratio of 5 to 1, but most people consume significantly more omega-6. Therefore, it makes sense to pay more attention to the intake of omega-3. Particularly rich in omega-3 are linseed oil and flaxseed, walnuts and fatty fish, for example salmon and herring. However, it is healthier to get your omega-3 from plant sources, as these contain more unsaturated fatty acids and animal sources usually contain more saturated fatty acids.

Fatty acids can also be divided into cis and trans forms. Trans fatty acids are harmful to the body, they have been proven to promote, for example, coronary heart disease and lipometabolic disorders. The best known example of the formation of trans fatty acids is the hydrogenation of fats, which is mainly used in the production of margarine. It is also suspected that trans fats are formed when oils are heated several times, which is why frying fat should never be used more than once.

## CARBOHYDRATES, FATS AND PROTEINS IN THE RIGHT MEASURE

Now we have brushed off the three most important macromolecules in relation to nutrition. I hope I didn't bore you too much with the chemical basics. But I didn't want to skip it because I think everyone should have heard about it at least once, especially, of course, people who are trying to eat healthier. A deeper understanding of our food and the substances that make it up helps immensely.

Lastly, I would like to address one more important topic. It is not only important to consume carbohydrates, fats and proteins in a healthy form, but also to distribute them properly. How many calories a person should eat a day depends on gender, age, activity, height, weight and other factors. If you wish, you can calculate this exactly on certain Internet sites. As a rough guide, however, you can take about 2000 kcal per day.

Don't get me wrong, this is not about losing weight. It's about a healthy lifestyle, which also depends on the number of calories we eat every day. Cardiovascular diseases, such as heart attacks, strokes and coronary heart disease, are the number one cause of death in Germany. Major risk factors for such diseases are obesity and diabetes. In the case of leaky gut syndrome, too, we now know that a healthy diet is an important component of therapy.

So, now back to our 2000 kcal per day. These 2000 kcal should consist of a certain amount of carbohydrates, proteins and fats. Again, it depends on factors such as gender and activity, but we again take the rough guide value for illustration. This assumes about 265 grams of carbohydrates, 65 grams of fat and 75 grams of proteins per day. Most people consume far too little protein, but a lot of fat and, above all, many quickly digestible carbohydrates. As a result, the feeling of hunger comes back much faster after the meal and we consume more (unhealthy) calories at the end of the day than would be good. There are many apps that allow you to determine your calorie goal and grams of macromolecules per day individually based on height, weight and so on. You can then enter into the app what you ate throughout the day. You can do this manually by looking at the nutrition table on the back of the food, but also easily with a barcode scanner using your phone's camera.

Of course, there is absolutely nothing wrong with not arriving at the exact values. These values serve as orientation and may also be exceeded or undershot from time to time. If you simply try to stick to them approximately, that is already a big step in the right direction. Looking a little more often at the nutritional value table of the foods you often buy and eat will also give you a feeling over time for how much added value a food brings you. I don't know about you, but I used to not be able to do anything at all with the values in this table. A nut bar with 3 grams of protein and 16 grams of carbohydrates - what is that supposed to tell me now?

# In summary: 6 steps to treat a leaky gut.

1. track your nutritional behavior, the easiest way to do this is via an app. This way you can also see in retrospect which foods you have eaten and how your body has reacted to them. You should try to avoid foods that increase or do not improve your symptoms.

2. Eyes open when buying food! If you have noticed that industrial sugars aggravate your symptoms, you should carefully check the food in the supermarket. This may take some time at first, but over time you will get to know the different foods better. Pay particular attention to paraphrased names for certain foods; for example, maltose and sucrose are also names for sugar.

3. Reduce stress - easier said than done, I know. In the associated chapter, I explained in detail what resilience is and why stress can be so unhealthy for us. Reducing stress or learning to deal with it properly is a process. Every person can positively influence his or her method of dealing with stress. It is possible, just not overnight. Take your time and don't be too hard on yourself.

4. Fight the cause, not the symptoms. Symptomatic treatment will alleviate the symptoms for a short time, but it is not a permanent solution for a symptom-free life. There are detailed tips on this in the chapter "And what can I do myself now?". If remedying the cause should not show any relief in your case, please do not be afraid to use medication after medical clarification.

5. Since the symptoms of leaky gut syndrome are quite nonspecific and varied, there are other diagnoses that have the same symptoms but have a completely different cause and thus require different therapy. Thus, when diagnosing leaky gut syndrome, it is essential to rule out the differential diagnoses. Differential diagnoses include irritable bowel syndrome and histamine intolerance.

6. Changing your diet doesn't work overnight, because it takes time to notice the positive effects. So that you don't lose the fun in the matter and remain consistent, it is important not to forbid yourself anything. Even with a change in diet, it's okay to eat unhealthy foods now and then.

# Closing words

One of the most important aspects of changing your diet is to remain constant and develop responsible eating habits. There is no point in banning yourself from certain foods. This may work for two or three weeks, but not permanently. If we forbid ourselves something, we only get more desire for it. In addition, the positive purpose of the change is overshadowed by the negative aftertaste of a strict renunciation. It is not at all bad to drink alcohol or eat sugar from time to time, this will neither kill you nor ruin all the successes of the dietary change so far. If you have learned to observe your body and its reaction to different foods, you will quickly realize that a certain amount of unhealthy food will not cause a bad reaction.

Finally, it is also very important for me to say that you should look for a doctor with whom you feel well cared for. Nonspecific complaints, such as concentration problems, fatigue, diarrhea or abdominal pain, are often misjudged and dismissed as irrelevant. However, if such complaints occur permanently, this is definitely not normal and the cause should be eliminated. There is no reason to have to deal with permanent complaints that are actually treatable.

Both in medicine and in psychology, there is the term "bias", which can be roughly translated as "thinking error". In the medical context, bias refers to the phenomenon that we subconsciously discriminate against some people for a wide variety of reasons, for example on the basis of their gender, skin color or religion. As a result, the complaints of the person concerned are perceived in a distorted way by the doctor. For example, women are stereotypically attributed with being more sensitive and sensitive to pain than men. As a result, painkillers are prescribed less frequently for women. Symptoms such as constipation and abdominal pain or abdominal cramps are also often subject to errors in thinking and explained away as period complaints - and without a thorough investigation into the causes of the complaints. If you feel that you are not being taken seriously with your complaints, you should seek treatment from someone else. Do not let yourself be persuaded that it is normal to always have problems with your bowels.

www.ingramcontent.com/pod-product-compliance
Lightning Source LLC
Chambersburg PA
CBHW051310160726
47994CB00003B/1403